Discovering & Treating the Facet Syndrome

Case Studies for 12 Medical Specialties

Discovering & Treating the Facet Syndrome

Case Studies for 12 Medical Specialties

By Nikolaos Giantsios
Orthopaedic Surgeon

WTM News Limited

2014

First Printing: 2014

ISBN 978-0-9927821-0-8

Author
Nikolaos Giantsios

Editor & Producer
Konstantinos Giantsios

Published by
WTM News Limited
Office 4, 219 Kensington High Street,
Kensington, W8 6BD, United Kingdom
www.wtmnews.com

Dedication

This book is dedicated to my wife and children.

Contents

Disclaimer

The information provided in this book is designed to provide helpful information on the subjects discussed, encourage medical practitioners to consider additional potential causes of medical symptoms and researchers to expand the scope of their research into adjacent medical domains. The information provided here presents an analysis and interpretation of personal experiences and under no circumstances does it constitute the result of formal research or a guide of any kind.

This book is addressed strictly to qualified practitioners only and is not meant to be used nor should it be used, to diagnose or treat any medical condition. The author warns practitioners and researchers that many of the ideas presented here require a high level of expertise and may hide significant risks. Medical practitioners are strongly advised to seek expert advice on any issues that exceed their education, training, experience and expertise. For diagnosis or treatment of any medical problem, patients are strongly advised to consult their own physician.

The publisher and author are not responsible for any health issues that may require medical supervision and are not liable for any damages or negative consequences from any treatment, action, application or preparation, to any person reading or following the information in this book. The publisher and author are not responsible for any issues that might arise as a result of actions taken by a person reading or following the information in this book.

About the Author

Nikolaos (Nikos) Giantsios was born in Thessaloniki in 1932 and was brought up in Kozani, the home town of his parents.

He received his degree from the Medical School of Thessaloniki University. His postgraduate training as an Orthopaedic surgeon lasted a total of six and a half years; eighteen months in Athens (Children Orthopaedic Hospital of Penteli)and five years through six hospitals in the United Kingdom including Royal National Orthopedic Hospital, Chesterfield Royal Hospital, War Memorial Hospital (Rhyl, North Whales), Oswestry Hospital, South Mead & Cossham Memorial Hospitals (Bristol) and Burnsley Hospital.

He has been practicing Orthopaedics in Thessaloniki since 1967. During this period he held appointments as a Consulting Orthopaedic Surgeon at the 1st Surgical University Clinic in AHEPA hospital from 1967 to 1976 and later at the Theagenio Cancer Hospital from 1979 to 1986. From that time onwards, he was confined strictly to private practice.

He did that mainly to reduce his workload and have more family time. He has two grown up children, Konstantinos and Fotini, for which he is very proud. He stopped skiing at the age of 78 when his wife Olga wisely refused to follow him down the red & black slopes any longer. Now he enjoys hiking and gardening with her. Carpentry is always a hobby and a passion. He strongly believes that a few glasses of wine go a long way towards enriching and livening up a productive conversation.

Preface

When the mechanisms of automation in the human body are in trouble the result is morbid manifestations, often appearing as clinical entities of obscure aetiology. These can in a surprising number of cases be enlisted as facet syndromes since they respond to treatment when treated as such. They involve a wide range of medical specialties in addition to orthopaedics.

The diagnosis of these syndromes is difficult since the channels used belong to the autonomous nervous system. The latter, guarding its secrecy, is unwilling to provide information to the examiner. What it allows to be revealed is hardly an invitation to solve a puzzle.

Once the association between the symptoms and the facets is suspected, then the local injections are those who can verify this. The author hereby presents a plethora of such cases involving 12 medical specialties. They all have been treated successfully and repeatedly, the same way, over his 45 year career.

Using the term facet syndromes, the author refers to a series of clinical entities which are caused when fine nerve endings, located in the capsule of the spinal facet joints, are in trouble. Similar sensors are also found in muscles, tendons and articular capsules of other joints. These sensors provide information about posture and gravity forces, most essential information for the kinetic and balance system. The irritation of these proprioceptors is the triggering mechanism for the appearance of these syndromes.

It is these clinical entities which doctors of various medical specialties very often come across and are called to treat. The inability to diagnose them as cases, whose origin is the spinal column, is what makes their treatment difficult.

Cases of this kind concern dentists, stomatologists, ENT surgeons, ophthalmic surgeons, general surgeons, gastro-enterologists, neurologists, neurosurgeons, urologists, gynecologists, cardiologists and chest specialists. To the orthopaedic surgeons belongs the major share of these syndromes although they do not suspect it.

The spinal origin of these syndromes was found at the beginning accidentally while treating patients with painful spinal conditions using the PVI (Para Vertebral Injections), a treatment technique with which he is familiar. Patients treated this way, often reported back stating that other clinical conditions from which they were also suffering for some time and seemed to be irrelevant to their present problem, were also cured or showed significant improvement.

This unexpected outcome of the treatment they had, was in effect trespassing, a crossing of the boundaries between medical specialties. Not surprising, patients belonging to these ill-defined areas are prone to meet difficulties when they have to decide who the right specialist to treat them is. A very significant number of these cases the author considers to be spinal facet syndromes and they should be treated as such.

What is common with theses clinical conditions is that the aetiology is obscure and their treatment consequently difficult. One can hardly detect any affinity with the spine. Most of them can present themselves at times with a different clinical picture that refers to a different medical specialty. As a result, wrong diagnosis and treatment is not uncommon with all the associated financial and social consequences following.

This book is addressed to doctors of almost all medical specialties. The author invites his colleagues to rediscover this part of medicine believing that his approach to certain medical conditions could serve as more effective alternatives to existing treatments. The thoughts and views presented here, do not represent the results of a formal medical research process, but a practitioner's personal experience as he systematically explored this domain over the past 45 years.

The reader is encouraged to be inquisitive into the contents of this book and is reminded of the fact that quite frequently, what one considers as experience is nothing more than the repetition of wrong ideas adopted and practiced over time until effective alternatives are discovered.

The questions which arise, further to what the author believes, should be discussed and answered by the medical specialties involved. The author, a trespasser in fields of foreign medical jurisdiction himself, would be the last one to do this. Further, the reader is alerted that the treatment techniques discussed here hide significant dangers which only highly trained and experienced professionals could be in the position to handle.

Introduction

The treatment of orthopaedic cases with medication delivered through the oral or intramuscular route proves quite often to be inadequate in bringing the desirable results. Early in my career, when I started using the local injecting technique, things became much easier for quite a number of cases. With this I could provide locally sufficient medication to the suffering area saving the rest of the body from undesirable side effects. My postgraduate training in United Kingdom gave me the opportunity to get familiar with this technique.

Upon my return to Greece, I started to apply on the cervical spine what I had learned to do on the lumbar one. Gradually I discovered that I could treat conditions which doctors of other medical specialties to whom they traditionally belonged to could not deal with, simply because they would not associate the symptoms to a spinal cause. With time and continuously on the lookout for similar cases, I realized that quite a number of medical specialties had similar problems. Many years later, when the facet syndrome was first described, I came to realize that what I was treating all these years was nothing else other than facet syndrome cases. With this term we refer to various clinical conditions which are the result of irritation of the nerve sensors, the proprioceptors, which are encountered in the capsule of the spinal facet joints.

Much later I came to realize that orthopaedic surgeons had the same difficulties since many of their obscure diagnostic problems are facet syndromes too. Funny enough, I came to this conclusion long after finding out what was happening with the other specialties. This is probably due to the fact that bone change caused by a bone infarct or another cause is not detectable at an early stage on the ordinary X-R films. Today MRI reports detect from the start blood supply interference and impending or established bone necrosis. They cannot verify a reversible or permanent intraosseous vascular change neither to confirm if there are still bone cells alive or not. Furthermore, they cannot point out any connection with the facets. The diagnosis of a facet syndrome in my days was purely clinical and I believe it still is.

The medical specialties which apart from orthopedics can be victims of facet interference are dentistry, stomatology, ENT surgery, neurology, neurosurgery, ophthalmology, gastroenterology, urology, cardiology, general surgery and chest specialty if such one exists.

All cases reported here belong to the above mentioned specialties. The decision to classify them as facet syndromes was based on the fact that they could be cured only when the facets were treated first. For organization purposes, an informal classification has been applied according to the location of the related facets on the spine. The interpretations given while discussing each case were inevitable. Nature hates vacuum and so does our mind.

This book is not the result of a formal medical research process but merely a presentation of my personal experiences, my interpretation of certain challenging medical conditions and the treatment techniques that I have found most beneficial to the patients and even myself, as they all matured in my mind over my 45 year career as an Orthopaedic Surgeon. I have chosen to use an informal way of presenting my ideas and I am confident that in the following pages you will find plenty of food for thought.

The Start of My Journey

February 1962 found me in London at the Royal National Orthopaedic Hospital, the teaching hospital of the British Orthopaedic Institute, attending a three month training course as a post graduate student. My previous experience in orthopaedics was 18-month training as an SHO (Senior House Officer) in a Children's Orthopaedic Hospital in Athens.

This was the start of an Odyssey through six hospitals in Britain. The British education system at the time, demanded from doctors to move from hospital to hospital up to the end of their training. The appointments of SHOs lasted one year, while those of Registrars a maximum of two. In other words, the British applied in education what Homer wrote 3.000 years ago in Odyssey (*"he visited the cities of many people and understood their way of thinking"*), in order to point out what he really believed to be the source of Ulysses' wisdom.

The training consisted of attending lectures, ward rounds, theater operations and outpatient clinics. The admitted patients were nursed usually in common wards and attended by the same nursing and medical stuff, while the junior medical stuff attended patients of more than one consultant. The consultants, representing the British Orthopaedic Institute, were as expected to be among the most eminent. Their approach to orthopaedic problems was quite often different. In lectures as well as in practice, they strived to be pioneers.

What they were really doing was searching for new ideas that would provide better solutions to everyday problems. This was actually the start of the most interesting period in my career as an orthopaedic surgeon, realizing that absolute knowledge does not exist. In fact, I realized that no one could hand down omniscient experience and instead I had to build up my education without the luxury of adopting ideas and practices unchallenged.

This actually started in May 1962 with my first appointment as an SHO at the Royal Hospital in Chesterfield, a small town of Derbyshire in the Midlands. The orthopaedic clinic was a relatively small one with 45 beds, two consultants, one registrar and one SHO.

It is evident that in a reverse pyramid system like this, all the supporting work was shared between the Registrar and the SHO in a way that a heavy week of 127 hours was followed by a lighter one of 96. Our abilities were rewarded by being offered more responsibility.

The fifth month, the senior consultant E.A.Nicoll, asked me to take over the Injection Clinic. Every Wednesday, between 2pm and 5 pm a number of 15 to 25 outpatients with joint and spinal problems would be looked after. The para vertebral injections (P.V.I.) to the lower spine, was common practice in England that time. I was given the proper instructions and left alone to my own devices. This continued for the next seven months until the end of my appointment.

As an experience I found it terrific. It was quite a challenge to get familiar in approaching almost any part of the skeleton with a needle, blindly, without any technical localizing aid. With the help of two well-trained nurses to pass syringes and prepare the next patient before the previous one was done, an average of 7-8 minutes was enough for each patient, including a brief questioning.

Each patient was reporting back in a week's time for his second injection, if so required. From that moment on, the clinic's patient automatically became my patient too, since his improvement lied in my hands. The possible negative result demanded an answer and there were two possibilities: wrong diagnosis or wrong selection of the area to be injected. I admit that the answer is far from being easy. It took me many years to figure it out.

The idea behind infiltrations is similar to the notion of watering the plant instead of the field, which is the problem with the usual administration of drugs. With local injections, the treated area receives adequate medication, since the locally acting preparation of cortisone is lasting for at least one week and the amount that is absorbed to the general circulation is negligible and harmless. It is practically the treatment of choice for patients whose stomach, liver and kidneys, don't welcome drastic medication.

My next job in orthopaedic training, after a six month interval of training in general and vascular surgery at Burnsley, was in Rhyl, a nice small town of North Wales. Consultant was Robert Owen, an excellent surgeon, clinician and teacher.

Actually he is the one who introduced me to new ideas concerning conditions that might be influenced by the spine. One out of many that I remember is that he considered tennis elbow to be related with the A6 level. At the time, besides being in charge of the orthopedic department of the War Memorial hospital in Rhyl, he was also Director of Studies at Oswestry and a few years later he was appointed Professor of Orthopaedics in Liverpool.

Since then, whenever I came across a painful peripheral syndrome I examined the spine for a possible participation, as a predisposing factor. My explanation at the time was that peripheral joints, ligaments, tendon sheaths, muscular insertions etc. can develop some sort of neurogenic, non-septic, inflammation after strain or minor trauma, when the spine suffered in some way.

The next two years I had the opportunity to practice PVI at Oswestry and later in Bristol where as a Registrar at Southmeed hospital, being in charge of my own outpatient clinic, I had to decide myself which treatment would be best for my patients.

Upon returning to Greece in1967, I was appointed Consultant Orthopedic Surgeon at the A' Surgical University Clinic, at the AHEPA Hospital of Thessaloniki. At the time, trauma was treated by General Surgeons, as it was customary in England many years ago and the appointment of bone and vascular specialists was crucial, especially when heavy trauma had to be dealt with.

The only existing Orthopaedic Hospital in Macedonia (the northern district of Greece), was in Kilkis, a small town 70km from Thessaloniki, where apart from trauma, cold cases were mainly treated. The AHEPA Hospital was a purely university hospital. Gradually and unofficially I turned to be the consulting orthopaedic surgeon to the other five university clinics; two of Internal Medicine, the Pediatric clinic, Neurology and the Neurosurgery clinics. Occasionally my services were offered to the neurosurgeons when unstable fractures of the cervical spine required surgical stabilization. Facing combined problems over a period of nine years with colleagues of different departments, had certainly an impact on my approach to medicine.

Working with general surgeons, I had the opportunity to extend my injecting experience to the cervical spine. The outpatient clinics were crowded with patients suffering from persisting post-traumatic pain. Treating the whiplash injuries was most gratifying. The injecting technique was extended to almost all cases of cervical syndromes since quick results were obtained.

My appointment to the Cancer Hospital brought me to close collaboration with oncologists, hematologists and urologists. Having gained the reputation of being able to cure headaches and other persisting neuralgias, all sorts of patients swarmed to me hoping of finding a solution to their chronic problem.

As I was nearing the end of my career, the main bulk of work was injection treatments. The cases which will be discussed, here, are just a representative sample out of a number of cases which I grossly calculate to be a lot more than 5.000. More than 60% of them had to do with the spine.

Myths & Theories

Quite a lot has been written lately about the so called "Cervical Facet Syndrome." This includes most of what we meant in the past by the term "Cervical Syndrome" and other post traumatic conditions. This confines as origin of various symptoms the articular capsule of the posterior articulations of the vertebrae, mainly those of the cervical spine.

The articular capsule of the posterior vertebral joints, is the host of a rich plexus of very fine neural fibers whose sensors, the proprioceptors, provide information to the labyrinth, the balance center of the loco-motor system, about posture, gravity forces etc. These proprioceptors are present also in tendons, muscles, ligaments and capsules of other joints. They are doing the same job as those of the facets. Inwards information arrives to this center from other sensory systems too, like vision and hearing which are also "online". This implies that when in trouble and at any given time these sensors have open channels of communication to send a distress signal to any direction. Trauma and mechanical strain are usually the reasons that upset them.

The balance center, vision and hearing centers as well the motion center are the receivers of these signals. Their vasomotor centers can be stimulated resulting to spasms of the nutrient vessels to nerves and organs or a vasomotor inflammation at a later stage. This implies that ENT surgeons and ophthalmologists might encounter problems too. This concept helped explain conditions I had by coincidence come across.

I will try to explain what I mean by open channels. Let us take the example of a football player. When he is training, the continuous repetition, improves skillfulness and tackling tactics which are stored in memory available to be drawn out on demand. In action, he does not have to improvise anything. The brain cortex decides which dexterity is best for that moment. The perfection of his performance has been already decided earlier during his practice. The sensors of the facet joints provide information about his stance and gravity. They are there ready to help him when he loses his balance and to let him understand his limits. Vision and hearing function in the same way.

This information flow is continuous. It starts from the periphery with a direction to the center and stops only in a black out or when at sleep. When a facet joint is injured, the sensors suffer too. They have no difficulty sending distress signals for help. The routes of communication are already open to them. Their duty is normally to report to the centers above them all the information they grasp. Now they are reporting at their own hazard.

Distress signals have now reached the headquarters of the autonomous nervous system. The latter being an inferior center, has no authority to take any action. Communication language between them and the supreme authority, which is the cortex, does not exist. When smoke signals are ignored by the cortex, what remains to the inferior centers to do is to proceed even with sacrifices. This is now what the vasomotor centers are asked to do.

This inability of direct communication between the autonomous system and the cortex should not be taken as a weakness. It may be that this is the secret to our survival. If we imagine the autonomous system as the civil service or the administration of a state, then what guards its integrity from the corruption of the politicians or the cortex, is the precise lack of direct liaison.

As one can suspect, attempting to organize in categories cases whose scope spans across medical domains, is not possible. For the purposes of this book I have grossly classified them into two groups. The first is related to the cervical area and the second to the lumbar one. This does not imply that the facets who are responsible belong to the corresponding spinal area exclusively. May be this is true in the majority of cases but not always. A headache for example of spinal origin could be quite often related to lumbar facets and possibly, although rarely, to proprioceptors of distal joints.

More than one medical specialty can be involved in the clinical picture. The facet proprioceptors whose privilege is to have all communication channels open and at their disposal, can send distress signals to many receptors at a time which in turn cause symptoms addressed to more than one specialty.

The possible recipients in the first group could be orthopaedic surgeons, neurologists, neurosurgeons, dentists, ENTs, ophthalmic surgeons, cardiologists, gastroenterologists and chest specialists. The recipients of the lumbar facets cases, in addition to the orthopaedic surgeons are the general surgeons, urologists, gynecologists, gastroenterologists etc.

There is no clear distinction between these two groups, since the facets, no matter how remote they are from the central nervous system theoretically they have equal chances of access to any vasomotor center belonging to any collaborating system. In this sense, although the cervical facets are those who can usually cause a headache, nobody can exclude proprioceptors from a knee joint to do the same.

In a relapse the same facets may attack a different system each time and cause a different clinical picture. The confusion starts with the patient himself when he picks the specialist he believes to be the right one to solve his problem.

Cervical Area

Dentists, ENT Surgeons, Neurologists

Let me start with a case where the dentist was the one to whom the ball was thrown first. This happened 25 years ago and concerns a woman, age 40, operator of a sewing machine. On the phone, she asked me if I had any idea about sinuses. Although my reply was that sinuses don't belong to the orthopaedics field, she insisted on seeing me because she was told that "I cure headaches".

Her problem was pain, starting from the occiput, extending to the teeth anteriorly, day-in day-out for three years. At the beginning and in an attempt to help her, her dentist removed one by one all the teeth from the affected side, both upper and lower jaw, trying to find the one tooth that caused the pain. With her problem persisting, she then visited an ENT surgeon who diagnosed sinusitis which should be operated. The operation did not help her at all. With the pain persisting, she visited a second ENT surgeon, who also diagnosed sinusitis and suggested a second operation for a better curettage, which she accepted but still without the anticipated result.

I told the patient that I had no idea about teeth or sinuses. Yet, I accepted to examine her. Palpating her cervical spine and sensing tenderness, I felt that it was worth trying an injection. I explained to her that it was possible that her cervical spine was the source of her problems. The only way to find out was by injecting her neck.

In her despair she accepted my proposal at once, just as she had done before with my other colleagues and in fact said "That's why I am here doctor." I asked her to return in a week's time only if the injection would help her.

She never reported back but after eight months she returned asking for another injection. She was completely relieved from pain during all this time. The last few days she felt some vague pain that reminded her of the past nightmare and came back running to prevent living it through again. Five years later, she brought her mother-in-law for a problem in her spine. The last time that I saw her was a few years ago when she visited and asked advice concerning osteoporosis. Luckily, the cervical spine had never been a problem again in the last twenty five years.

There are some facts about this medical case, which should be discussed. First of all, the disappearance of the pain after injecting the facets confirmed that the problem was spinal. When I injected her neck, I suspected that it might help her but I was not sure. When the patient eight months later, told me that the pain had completely disappeared just with that one injection, this was something that I really could not understand. I could not figure out any possible mechanism through which the injection could work. Only years later did I realize that what I treated was a cervical facet syndrome, but the question of how the injection had worked was still not clear to me. A satisfactory answer came many years later. I will return to this later when I discuss headaches.

In regards to the dentist and the ENT surgeons, it is obvious that they did not suspect that the problem was a complex one. No matter how good they were, they could not have known something about which nothing had been written until then. The vasomotor reaction which the spine had produced in the area could easily have deceived both. They both had a local problem in their own territory which they could not ignore. None of them could say it is not my problem since everything they were touching was painful. They were in effect trapped.

If I had seen the patient first, before the dentist and the ENT surgeons, and if I had the experience that I have today I would still be unable to decide straight away under which specialty the case should be enlisted. I would now certainly try an injection and expect the answer to follow. This is what really happens when treating facet syndromes. You cannot ever have a single objective diagnostic proof of their existence. The answer to your hypothesis will only come the week after.

My experience in this subject has been acquired mainly from patients in despair who were approaching me for a possible solution, after others had failed. They all knew about my injections and were prepared to try them. They would never come first to me as they could not possibly imagine that an orthopaedic surgeon might help them with their problem. This is more or less what happened in almost all the cases which follow.

A few years ago, I was visited by a female patient around 65 years old, for a persisting brachial neuralgia. Over the previous few years she had all sorts of pain around the shoulder girdle and head. When I asked her if she ever had any problem with her teeth, she paused for a few seconds and then she asked me what I meant. I did not clarify my question further, so she said that the previous year she had two teeth extracted. The dentist, for whom she had been working as an assistant for twenty years, confessed to her that both extracted teeth were completely healthy.

Quite probably, the neuralgia which I diagnosed and cured as a facet-one had made its presence felt a year earlier as a dental neuralgia which could have probably been treated by injecting the facets instead of searching for the bad tooth.

The next case is presented just to show how difficult it can be for the patient to decide herself which specialist is the right one to help her. This is the case of a woman round 70. The patient felt something to snap in her cervical spine, while cutting to pieces the fourth quince in preparation of a special dish, as she pressed the knife hard on both its ends. Ignoring the incident, a few hours later she felt an acute causalgia in her tongue and an acute pain in her ear. Non-steroids helped for causalgia to subside after the fourth day.

The ENT surgeon told her that there was nothing wrong with her ears. The neurologist pointed to her that her cervical spine was probably the source of her problem. The tenth day, with the ear pain persisting she came to me.

At this point I must add that the patient was a trained nurse. I had injected her cervical and lumbar spine in the past. The symptoms of her recent problem were so fulminant that it did not cross her mind that her cervical spine could be the cause.

Five minutes after injecting her cervical spine the pain of the ear had disappeared and she could now raise her arm as she said. She did not dear do it before. She hadn't even mentioned it earlier as a symptom. The patient is usually incapable to suspect that a causalgia or an ear pain could be a referred skeletal symptom when aggravated just by lifting the arm or stretching the neck.

ENT Surgeons, Neurologists, Gastroenterologists

The next example concerns a woman, round 50 years old, with a serious swallowing problem. Her husband, a lawyer, rang me in despair to ask me if I knew anybody who could possibly help her. The ENT surgeon, the neurologist and gastroenterologist could not help. Her condition had been deteriorating continuously for two months.

I had seen the patient a couple of years earlier for a problem in her cervical spine and I suggested to see her myself first. When I examined her again, I noticed some tenderness of the muscles around her neck. I told her that I could try an injection to the spine as I had also done in the past. The only thing I could promise was that in the very least the injection could do no harm. One week later, her husband rang me to say that his wife was almost back to normal and asked for a second injection. He wanted to make sure that they would not live again the nightmare of death from starvation due to her acute swallowing problem. Up to this day she is still symptomless. Three more cases with dysphagia, similar to this, had a sensitive cervical spine and were treated in the same way with the same success.

Dysphagia is a problem of other specialties. It is quite natural, that nobody should expect from an orthopaedic surgeon to have any opinion on its aetiology. In a few dysphagia cases however cervical facets could be involved. The above mentioned cases responded to facet infiltration only.

One of these dysphagia cases, an elderly man round 70, returned a few months later with a facial neuralgia. There was numbness over his left cheek and upper lip, plus the typical facial paresis. At the time, still disciplined to the segmental distribution of pain and not having yet adopted my later beliefs of how the cervical facets might behave, it did not cross my mind to inject again his spine. He ended up with perforation of his cheek, as I was told. To this day, I still do not know if this was too, a different manifestation of a facet syndrome. What is certain, is that I lost the chance to find out and further more to help my patient.

I hope that the reader understands that many of the examples given in this book have always intrigued me testing the limitations of classic medicine. In the previous case there would be no questioning if the neurologists could have an answer.

The following case is another example that puzzled me. A patient of mine, whose neck I had injected the previous day, rang me to say that he got hiccups which started a few hours after the injection. The neuralgia was gone. It was quite natural for him to worry now if this was something that could be expected and for how long it would last. A light sedative helped a lot.

The first thing I thought, was that playing the needle up and down I had somehow traumatized the capsule of a facet joint which had in some way access to the diaphragm. I must admit that the next time I come across persistent hiccups I would be strongly tempted to inject the cervical spine, to find out if the reverse could happen. That said seeking answers in this way is something I would never advise others to do! It is like accelerating on a slippery road.

Chest Specialists, Neurologists, Cardiologists

I will continue with a few more examples, just to cover the area of the remaining specialties where facets can get involved.

This is the case of a doctor, friend of mine with an irritable cough. The lung specialist could not find anything to justify it. A few weeks later he presented a brachial neuralgia which perplexed both neurologists and neurosurgeons. When he came to me he was almost convinced that he had some sort of obscure lung cancer with a metastasis to the spine. Injecting the cervical spine, hopping to cure neuralgia, the cough disappeared too.

Another female patient age around 70 now, whom I have been treating from time to time over the last thirty years, confessed to me lately that when sometime in the past I had injected her neck, a persisting cough had also stopped.

This same patient came to me once with a brachial neuralgia. Feeling her pulse, I diagnosed a cardiac arrhythmia. There was a pause after every three or four normal pulses. Mentioning this to her she protested saying that the cardiologist, whom she had visited a few days ago, had told her that cardiac function was checked to be completely normal. The next day, after having injected her neck, both neuralgia and arrhythmia were gone. I thought that this was the sort of arrhythmia which the cardiologists call "out-cardiac" and they do not seem to worry much about.

Cases of acute dizziness, especially after turning or extending the neck are those who respond dramatically to facet infiltration. The ENT surgeon usually cannot help. The only thing that connects him with this is the symptom.

Which areas can the facets affect?

The mucosa of the upper respiratory tract is a usual area where facet joints may cause a peripheral vasomotor inflammation. Congestion of mucosa can affect drainage of sinuses, cause unexplained chronic inflammations in this area, respiratory difficulties and so on. The first example which I mentioned earlier, proved to be a real problem of this kind for the dentist and ENT surgeon.

Some cases of unexplained painful conditions in the mouth could possibly also be related to facets, causalgia and mouth ulcerations being one of them.

A few of my patients had come seeking help for a relapse of trigeminal neuralgia that they had in the past. Their present problem was just a cervical facet syndrome, which responded after been treated as such. Not being familiar with this sort of clinical entity, I believed that they were confusing their present problem with what they had in the past. If what they had in the past was the same, then it was facet neuralgia.

If the neurologists are still in doubt today on the aetiology of this sort of neuralgia, now they can try to treat it on its onset as a facet syndrome. Who knows; that might be the answer. Some old standing cases of trigeminal neuralgia, years after their onset, did not respond to facet infiltrations. You cannot help when irreversible changes have been established.

A few years ago I was touring Syria with a group, of mostly Americans. One of them was suffering from sleep apnea. He had found solution to his problem with a CPAP device (Continuous Positive Airways Pressure). One morning, sitting in the internal garden of the hotel in Damascus, I was watching two men walking on the glass roof. "Look at them", I said addressing to him. He replied that he could not look upwards because he would feel dizzy. That moment I knew that he had a cervical facet syndrome. What I did not know was if the sleep apnea had anything to do with this too.

Internal Medicine, ENT Surgery & Ophthalmology

One day I met Ann, the English teacher of my children. Her husband Bill, a teacher too, had recently taken over the management of a private English teaching school and started to organize everything electronically. She was worried for him. The last few weeks he did not feel well. The doctors could not find any obvious reason, so they suggested admission to hospital for a checkup. I offered to see him.

The patient, a well-organized and hard working person, felt for the first time in his life, that something was wrong with him. Dizziness and slight instability were what worried him most. He attributed the stiffness of his neck to prolonged work on his PC. I told him that most probably he had put too much strain on his neck, which in turn reacted this way. We could easily find out if it was so by injecting his cervical spine. Because I had treated his mother-in-law in the past with injections and he had seen the results, he accepted it.

Three days later he rang me to say that he was back to normal. One thing he wanted me to explain to him. How was it possible to think more clearly, to hear and see better, even colors to be brighter? This dramatic improvement is characteristic for cases where symptoms have not lasted too long. This actually happens when peripheral organs vessels and nerves have not sustained yet irreversible changes. Treating the facets only is all they need.

Years later I ran again into his wife. She introduced me to her friend from London visiting her. Turning to her she said "this is the doctor I was telling you about last night who saved Bill six years ago with just one injection". This was an indirect confirmation that the injection had really helped him.

Ever since, I always questioned patients visiting me for problems related to the cervical spine, for any problems concerning vision and hearing. Some of them reported blurred vision, easy fatigue in reading and difficulty in focusing, for which the ophthalmologist could not find an obvious reason. They usually reported on our next appointment that in addition to their headache or neuralgia for which they had come, the ophthalmic symptoms had improved too.

Some of my patients, who had at times problems with their cervical spine, had a history of retinal detachment, after trivial injury to the head. I entertained myself to believe that facets could have possibly affected the retina to the point that a minimal trauma could produce a fissure to the retina. A myopic person exerts more mechanical stress to his cervical spine than any other person with normal vision, trying hard to focus at work, even when wearing glasses. May be this is a reason why they are more prone to detachment.

These kind of simplified and arbitrary interpretations were the result of my obsession, that the eyes could not possibly be immune from facet interference since vision is an indispensable partner in the function of the loco-motor system keeping open channels of communication with it.

Personal Case Study: My Olive Tree

I will continue with an example which concerns myself personally and happened a few years ago. I have a big olive tree in my garden that gives about eighty kilograms of olives every year. It took me three days to collect them one by one climbing on a ladder. I admired my stiff neck for not protesting. The third and last day, waking up after a short siesta, I realized that I was completely deaf from my left ear.

I remembered farmers visiting me after olive collection and tree pruning with similar symptoms. They were usually helped after injecting their spine. The ENT surgeon told me that he sees quite often cases of acute deafness. Some of them recover completely, some not. The aetiology is not clear. As far as treatment is concerned some prescribe vasodilating drugs, others heavy doses of cortisone. Knowing no one of my colleagues to practice para vertebral injections to the cervical spine, I took both types of medication. Which means my only choice was to water the field instead of just the one thirsty tree. The amount of cortisone I took was ten times more than that of the injection and the amount that reached the tree one hundredth. My hearing recovered by 30% only. The stereoscopic hearing was lost.

The example is clearly personal. It is well known that doctors are notorious of being unreliable when they have to diagnose themselves. The diagnosis of a facet syndrome is verified only by the result of treatment. In my case injection was not an option. So, adequate confirmation is missing. This report might be useful as a stimulus only for further research by those who care to investigate further.

In my case, the ENT surgeon had to treat a suffering organ and save nerve cells from dying. If my belief, that my case was a cervical facet syndrome is right then it sounds logic to think that injecting the facets one could help the ENT surgeon to do his job more effectively. By the moment the facets are properly attended to and happy, they have no reason to continue grumbling and force the vasomotor centers to perpetuate their interference.

I intend to continue with a second example which I believe to be related to my arthritic cervical spine. One day I woke up with a stiff neck and heavy head. The previous day, I had done heavy manual work exceeding my limits. My blood pressure which normally lies round 120/70 was found to be 170/105. Suspecting my facets to be protesting I took for one day only two tablets of a non-steroid anti-inflammatory drug, notorious for raising the blood pressure, in an effort to calm down the facets. Next day my blood pressure was almost back to normal.

I did a cross check with patients who under normal conditions their blood pressure was not exceeding the accepted limits. When I treated them for facet problems their raised blood pressure was not a contraindication to inject their spine. Actually their blood pressure improved. When I talked with cardiologists they had a hard time accepting the way I brought down my benign and transient hypertasis.

One day I had a visit from a female patient, age around sixty five. She had a problem in her cervical spine. I had the feeling that this was another facet syndrome and that my injections could help her. She told me that she was on treatment with steroids for five years now for temporal arteritis, and whatever treatment I decided, this should not interfere with the cortisone treatment she was on.

The reader can realize here a tricky situation between a patient, content with the diagnosis and treatment she was already on and an obsessed doctor who suspected a facet implication behind every obscure diagnostic problem. I decided not to treat her and I sent her for physiotherapy.

Her problem could have probably been treated by injecting her spine. The established arterial pathology could not be reversed. The injection of the spine however would probably be incriminated for any possible future problem concerning the eyes. If there is any relation between temporal arteritis and cervical facets, this is something that might concern the ophthalmologists to find out. If such a relation exists, then facets are those which should be blamed for a possible blindness. Temporal artery itself is just another "victim".

Headaches

Headaches are another thought-provoking subject. The experiences I had, relate to the cervical facets only. I felt completely incapable to help someone when the cortex was involved. Headaches related to cervical joints are those who can be dramatically improved after having the facets infiltrated with cortisone and xylocaine. My real problem was to understand how it worked in certain cases. It was inconceivable to accept that a single injection could cure a headache which had lasted for ten or twenty years. Only recently, while reading a paper written by an osteopath, I came up with what could be a possible explanation.

After an injury of a cervical joint, a muscular spasm follows that, in order to protect it from pain. This spasm immobilizes the spine in a convenient painless position which is probably what "locking" implies. If this immobilization continues for more than eight to ten days, it is sufficient time for adhesions to form between the adjacent surfaces of a capsular fold. A chiropractor, extending, flexing, rotating the spine to extreme positions and applying a carefully controlled jerk, does nothing more than to break these adhesions. Once this is done, the patient is relieved from pain.

Quite possibly, injecting the facets had the same effect. The only difference is that the manipulation was done not by me but by the patient himself, who, having been relieved from pain (this is what xylocaine achieved) tried instinctively to regain the lost range of movement. Further, the cortisone, with its anti-inflammatory action, prevented new adhesions to reform.

The following example illustrates the aforementioned point explicitly. This is about a village woman from a mountain village of Macedonia, age round sixty, who after losing her husband, looked after her few goats and cultivated her own garden. Her problem was a continuous headache that had lasted for more than ten years. I injected her neck and advised her to moderate the knitting she used to do after the end of a hard day's work. She would come again in case of improvement.

In ten days, keeping her appointment, she reported that the pain had completely gone. I pretended to be indifferent, and hiding my surprise, I asked her why she came back. Her answer was that she could not yet believe that a headache that had lasted for ten years could disappear so fast with just one injection. She probably came back to be reassured that this might not recur.

What I remember from her first appointment is seeing her, shortly after having injected her neck, turning her head to the left again and again, saying "Oh, I could not do this before".

It took me almost twenty years to realize that what she was actually doing there and then before my eyes was breaking adhesions. It was xylocaine that permitted this to happen and cortisone, which prevented new adhesions to reform. This is probably why the relief that the osteopath is achieving by manipulating the spine is quite often only temporary. Breaking the adhesions is practically a new trauma.

She was a straight forward character with no insecurities. Surviving day-by-day was the only thing that concerned her. Entering her house and closing the door behind her, meant leaving all her problems outside.

Sometimes one hears funny stories from his patients, which in reality are not funny at all. Once, one of my patients told me that he had a lasting headache in the past which started after a fall from his horse. Many years later, this pain disappeared abruptly after a second fall, from his tractor this time. I had reasons to believe he was not joking. If such was the case there should be an explanation and there was only one I could give. Quite probably the second injury had broken the adhesions which the first one had produced.

Now, there are headaches where injections cannot help. These are the cases where the cortex is involved. This was the case with another woman, also round 60 years old, who, trying to extend her flourishing women's clothing business she opened a second shop. She suddenly realized she had created financial problems she had not foreseen. These problems followed her everywhere. They could not be locked out. Injections would not help.

Most headaches related with the cervical spine have nothing to do with adhesions. It is the mechanical strain on cervical facets at work and injections can be effective only if the patient can adjust behavior and avoid further mechanical strain.

Facets & Segments; the Paradox

Considering that there is an on line communication of all the facet joints to the balance center, one has to accept that any one of them, no matter how remote it is, can have access to the system and can cause problems in unexpected areas. The segmental concept is something that the facets can ignore. The communication channels they use are different. I was led to this thinking treating patients with symptoms concerning both lumbar and cervical area. The following example is illustrating.

A woman, age 55, came with all sorts of pain round lumbar and cervical spine with radiation to head, arms and legs. She had her daughter's wedding in three weeks' time and was desperate for help to cope with her obligations. I told her that I could not inject both areas at a time and asked her which area to treat first. I injected the lumbar facets. Reporting back after one week she said that low back and legs improved a lot. What she could not understand was how all the pain from the cervical area was completely gone.

The minimal amount of cortisone that might have been absorbed to the general circulation, could not justify this dramatic effect. Segmental relation of lumbar facets with the cervical area does not exist. After this, whenever I came across a similar case, I suggested to start treating the lumbar spine first. This paradox of improvement of cervical problems by injecting just the lumbar facets was repeated in quite a number of cases. In all these cases there was no need to inject the cervical spine.

This paradox, of pain being relieved in areas which had no segmental relation to the injected facets, made me distrust at the beginning, the drug companies claiming that the action of their product was mainly local with minimal only and negligible absorption to the general circulation. I had the feeling that I was not quite sincere when I had to assure my patients that they should not be afraid of any side effects related to cortisone. This guilt complex followed me for almost two decades, even though I believed that the treatment I was offering was less harmful than any alternative one. This notion followed me until the time I came to suspect that the spinal facets were behind this paradox and not any absorbed amount of cortisone.

A relevant paradox is the following case which happened twenty to twenty five years ago. I used to recall it and be amused. It concerns a male patient about 50 years old with a medial periarthritis of his knee which remained in spite of the different treatments he had received. I proceeded to infiltration of all the tender area. I do not remember if I had injected his spine too. On next appointment he was happy to report that his knee was doing well. Before leaving my surgery he asked me if it was possible that the treatment he had received for his knee was the reason why he had got rid of a persisting headache of the last few weeks.

What at that time I accepted to be a coincidence and amused me, it later turned to be a puzzle and real headache, for me this time. If I would accept now in retrospect the possibility that the knee problem was related with his headache then it would be impossible for me to decide which proprioceptors were responsible. Was it those of the facets or those of the knee? What is certain now is that I cannot any longer be amused when I recall it.

At this point I have to mention some issues concerning the treatment. Once you diagnose a facet syndrome, this means that you accept that you are handling a mechanically induced disorder. It is some sort of injury in the past or mechanical strain in the present. Worn out facets are probably prone to react to mechanical stress. The injected cortisone will cure the inflammation. The patient himself has the responsibility to reduce the strain. You just throw the ball straight back to him. This explanation is done preferably at the next appointment, when he has already experienced some improvement. The patient will listen only if you have gained his confidence. The improvement he has felt is just the start of the healing process. There is no wound that heals in less than three weeks.

Lumbar Facets & Lower Extremities Cases

Pain around the trochanters and linea aspera, areas of insertion of the gluteal muscles, is usually some sort of local inflammation. The same is true for medial periarthritis of knees, tender heel, plantar fasciitis and arthritis along the medial border of the arch of the foot. In all of them a positive relation was found to exist between them and lumbar spine. The most common of them is the medial periarthritis of the knee or pes anserinus tendinitis. All require local infiltration no matter if the facets have been injected or not.

Pes anserinus syndrome?

(Idiopathic necrosis of medial femoral condyle and osteochondritis dissecans)

Eight or ten years ago, a woman known to be a fanatic mountaineer, came to see me, to get a second opinion. Two months earlier, she had visited a colleague for an arthralgia of her knee. The MRI reported evidence of impairment of the intraosseous blood supply of the medial femoral condyle.

Her doctor diagnosed an impending aseptic necrosis and she was submitted to some sort of expensive treatment, which lasted for seven to eight weeks. The treatment was aiming to save the bone cells by providing better oxygenation. A new MRI, eight weeks after the first one, did not show any improvement. The pain was the same and now the other knee had started bothering her too. Her doctor concluded that necrosis of the condyle was most probably established.

When I examined her, the clinical picture was that of a pes anserinus tendinitis. A definite tenderness was elicited too palpating the collateral side of her lumbar spine. She remembered that a low back pain was her problem for a period of a few months before her knee started hurting her.

Having the experience of previous cases, I told her that I could help her if she accepted, apart from the tender area of the knee, to have her spine injected too, though the spine did not bother her at the time. After two weekly sessions, the pain was gone. The MRI, done the third week showed complete restoration of the intraosseous circulation back to normal.

Although I have treated hundreds of cases of pes anserinus tendinitis, I am not familiar of how frequently the intraosseous blood supply of the medial femoral condyle is affected. One does not easily ask for x-rays, MRI or other examinations when treating a tendinitis or bursitis. The MRIs I have seen were those which my patients had already done before coming to me. They proved to be precious information.

A similar case follows. She was a patient round 60, with the same clinical picture of a pes anserinus tendinitis and the same MRI report of a probable medial femoral condyle necrosis. She had a history of 1st degree spondylolisthesis at the L4-L5 level and lately she had to climb stairs. She was treated the same way as the previous one. There was full clinical recovery and restoration of the MRI picture to normal after two sessions.

In both these two examples, the patients were diagnosed by me as lumbar facet syndromes and were treated as such. Both spine and knees were injected. The congestion of the femoral condyles subsided too in both cases. This has led me to think that quite possibly, what we call "idiopathic necrosis of medial femoral condyle", is nothing more than the end result of a lumbar facet syndrome which we have failed to diagnose and then treat it as such timely.

Osteochondritis dissecans was found to follow a pes anserinus syndrome on an elderly woman many months after its onset. At the beginning the problem was pain over the medial and posterior side of the knee and an oedema of the leg down to the foot. The sixth month she felt an acute snap in her knee while stepping down. Ordinary x-rays did not show any thing. The MRI revealed the necrosis at the central part of the weight-bearing part of the medial femoral condyle. Now the patient had a problem with the knee itself. Her doctor decided to drill the defect but he did nothing to help the tendinitis. Her condition was deteriorating.

The patient came to me one year after the onset of her problem, a few months after the drilling. The knee was swollen with fluid; there was 10 degrees loss of extension and the tenderness over the medial side of the joint still there. The patient had not any problem with her lumbar spine. What started the problem one year ago was the fact that she had to climb up and down 40 steps many times every day. This was enough of a reason to cause a pes anserinus tendinitis.

I felt that I had to treat both knee and periarthritis. The knee was aspirated and injected. The same was done to the tendon area. There was a dramatic relief of pain and disappearing of swelling of leg and ankle. The pain on weight bearing was minimal.

I dealt with the case considering this to be a pes anserinus syndrome and the tendon proprioceptors those who triggered the bone necrosis. There was no need for any lumbar facet proprioceptors to be involved. In this case an ordinary pes anserinus tendinitis, receiving no treatment evolved to a syndrome. It was the absence of any available effective treatment what has led to bone necrosis.

Many years ago, twenty or more, I met E.A. Nicoll, my previous consultant at Chesterfield, during one of his frequent visits to Greece. By that time I had collected more than one hundred cases of medial periarthritis of the knee, a condition, which was commonly called in England "cellulitis" or "bursitis" and was treated at the time with pericapsular injections, infiltrating the pes anserinus area. Most of my cases were women, rather obese with dilated superficial veins and in all of them there was a chronic problem of the lumbar spine. A perimalleolar oedema on the affected side was quite common.

I explained to him that my belief was that the spine was in some way responsible for this clinical entity since all these cases responded much better to treatment when, in addition to the local infiltration, the spine was injected too.

He showed to be interested. He told me he was at that time the editor of the Italian Orthopedic Journal. He offered to publish the paper provided he was the first to do it, it should be fully documented and I had to verify that nothing had been written before on the subject. He suggested that "pes anserinus syndrome" would be a good title.

I was really discouraged, realizing how difficult it was to proceed. The main reason was that I could not respond to the prerequisite of "full documentation". Most of my patients visited me for a second opinion. They were already examined before by other colleagues bringing with them all sorts of tests and x-rays that they previously were asked to do. These were their property which they carried away with them to be available for the next doctor that they might have to visit. All my patients were private and many of them would have to pay themselves for any further test I would ask.

If it will ever be decided pes anserinus tendinitis to have a place as a "syndrome" in orthopaedic literature, then the necrosis of the medial femoral condyle will lose its adjective "idiopathic", since its aetiology will be a known one, being the end result of an untreated pes anserinus syndrome.

Swollen ankles are certainly an aesthetic problem for women. This accompanies quite often this syndrome and they are pleased when they see that the perimalleolar oedema has subsided too while treating their knees.

I would like to make it clear that a tendinitis can exist without any facet involvement. If one has to go up and down stairs, especially circular and narrow with steps 20 cm high or higher, he can easily get a pes anserinus tendinitis which can easily heal with rest, even without medication. The vasomotor manifestations locally and in the vicinity diffuse radical pain. The persistence of pain in spite of rest and use of non-steroids is what makes the difference between a simple tendinitis and the syndrome.

Sudeck's Syndrome

Sudeck's syndrome (Reflex Sympathetic Dystrophy Syndrome - RSDS) is a clinical entity that concerns everyone who deals with trauma. It has been estimated that almost 5% of minor trauma and surgical intervention to upper and lower extremities are presenting this complication. It is a most painful and incapacitating clinical condition, some sort of non-septic local inflammation, affecting mainly the small joints of the extremities. Its social cost is enormous. The autonomous system is incriminated of being involved and surgeons have a really hard time trying to help.

Having preoccupied myself with the idea that persisting peripheral pain beyond an acceptable period could be related to the spine, in addition to the local problem, I had no hesitation to treat the spine too, in cases where there was evidence that the latter was involved. My feeling was that the trauma had possibly come in a moment when the spine already had its own problems. Treating both spine and peripheral problem, proved to be beneficial for my patients and certainly a great relief for me. When I gradually came to realize that what I was treating all these years was nothing else than facets, then the logical next step for me was to accept that Sudeck's osteodystrophy is just another facet syndrome. In addition to providing local relief, I was treating the cause of the problem. The success in handling these cases had nothing to do with any special dexterity.

During my training in England, almost fifty years ago, the frequency of persisting pain after treating a Colles' fracture in elderly ladies was quite a headache. It was irrelevant of how good the reduction and immobilization were. Quite often these patients were complaining about pain going up and down the arm and their most frequent complaint was that the cast was too heavy for them. By the time the cast was removed there was a painful oedema present, which made recovery most difficult.

Preoccupied with the idea that the spine might be responsible for the persistence of post traumatic or postoperative pain, causing some sort of neurogenic inflammation to the traumatized area, I had a close look on them during the period of immobilization. A history of cervical syndrome was an alarm going off, which could not be ignored. I used to prepare these restless patients saying that more difficulties might start the moment the cast is removed and in case mobility was not satisfactory by the end of the 1st weak out of plaster, a local infiltration might be needed.

Physiotherapy could help only after the oedema and pain subsided. I found it useful, in Colles' fractures, to change the cast by the end of the second week with a lighter one, in the neutral functional position, with the wrist in slight dorsal flexion, in order to start using the limb, while in cast. The use of a light acrylic cast proved to be precious at this stage. Informing my patients for things that might happen, they were prepared to follow whatever I suggested on the way to recovery and I could prevent the full development of the typical Sudeck's atrophy.

All the typical fully developed Sudeck's atrophy cases I had, were those which other colleagues had a really hard time to cope with and were quite happy to see them leave and visit another doctor. I must admit that I was happy to see them come to me since I had already classified them as spinal syndromes and I felt quite confident that I could cope with them. I will mention a few examples about cases which came to me in an advanced stage.

A desperate patient around 60 appeared one day asking for help. His left foot was swollen and bluish. He could not stand even the pressure of the bed sheet on it. All had started eight months ago after a sprain of his forefoot, during the move to another town. Recent x-rays showed an almost complete demineralization of tarsal and metatarsal bones. The previous colleagues, in spite of their efforts, were not very certain about the outcome and the patient was afraid that he was going to lose his leg. Physiotherapy of any kind had failed.

I told the patient that I would try a treatment with local injections. At the same time I should inject the spine too, because an irritable nerve, as I told him, did not permit the previous treatments to help him. This treatment would be repeated in a week's time only if this first one proved to be helpful. He reported back and had totally four more sessions of local infiltration. The lumbar spine was injected twice only. It took two weeks for the patient to attempt partial weight bearing. By the fifth week the physiotherapist took over. In three months the x-rays showed significant restoration of the bone density.

A second example concerns a woman, age 55, who had sustained an un-displaced Colles' fracture six months earlier. She did well after having the cervical spine and her wrist injected. Both radical pain and local tenderness subsided after three or four sessions. Some permanent stiffness of the wrist remained.

The third example is about a woman, age about 60, who sustained a crack fracture of lateral malleolus. She came to me the third month after injury. She did well in two sessions. After her recovery, she had to visit her previous doctor for a formality concerning her insurance. Stating that she had recovered, she avoided to mention my involvement. So her doctor called his colleagues to announce to them how effective, the last medicine he had prescribed, proved to be.

The only reason why I may have justification in mentioning that is the fact that Sudeck's syndrome is a nightmare for every orthopedic surgeon. It has also been for me in the past. I believe that frozen shoulder is a non-treated cervical facet syndrome. Vanishing bone is the end result of such conditions.

My reference to Sudeck's syndromes would be incomplete, if my treatment method is not also mentioned. I believed that all tender spots should be injected. If some of them could not be dealt with during the first appointment, because the patient could not tolerate any more pain, they should be done on the next one. The patient is ready to continue her treatment if she sees improvement. Treating these cases, it reminded me of the joke about somebody who insisted that he had discovered the ideal insecticide, "you just have to catch the insect, force its mouth open and drop the drug in it" he claimed. The analogy, treating bone atrophies, is that you have to inject every single tender small joint. It is not always necessary to inject the spine more than once when you have the feeling that the facets are calm. You do not need to draw the insect curtain when there are no mosquitoes around.

Injecting the facets only, you cannot cure a Sudeck's syndrome. Maybe they have started the problem by sending their distress signals to any direction, but the inflammation was created by the vasomotor centers, which took over after receiving the signals the facets had sent. Injecting the inflamed area I had the feeling that I was breaking a vicious circle. It was like putting a fire out. When the fireman does his job, he does not have to ask how things have started. His only problem is to find the most effective way to put it out.

Although this is how I dealt with orthopaedic problems of this kind since the late sixties, it was not until the nineties that I started formulating my ideas. I found facet syndrome, when it was first described, to be a wonderful scaffolding to build my own myths. I had no reason why I should not enlist Sudeck's bone atrophy among facet syndromes since I treated them successfully as such. I felt less of a heretic as far as my therapeutic approach is concerned and in fact really happy that I had not discovered anything new, so I did not have to give supporting evidence or prove anything to anyone.

I would like to close this chapter with one of my own cases. It was again a Colles' fracture. Removing the cast, it was obvious that there would be a difficult road ahead. The patient refused to have her wrist injected and her spine if required. She decided to try physiotherapy first. I saw her six months later, when she escorted her sister to my surgery. She was happy with her wrist which did not hurt anymore and was proud that she had the courage to struggle through thirty eight sessions of painful physiotherapy. The residual stiffness was something she hopped to overcome with time.

It is obvious that such a result was not a success. The cost in suffering, prolonged recovery, expenses and functional incapacity was quite heavy. Unfortunately, the facets, whose role is to serve fighters and acrobats, not cripples, cannot wait. They demand to be attended first.

Arthroplasties

The lasting of implants is of great concern to every surgeon. Although I believed in good technique and I accepted nothing less than perfect fitting of implants, regardless if cement was used or not, I do not think that this is enough. I had always been suspicious that spinal joints could play a role in the loosening of implants.

The analysis that follows is based on retrospect thinking, trying to understand why some arthroplasties lasted and others did not. At the time I had not developed any theory of how facets interfere. I just knew that injecting the posterior joints of the lumbar spine, I was relieving my patients from spinal symptoms. Using a needle 1 1/2" long, one cannot reach much deeper. Doing this, I probably stopped the facets from causing congestion and blood stagnation to the bones that hosted the implants.

To be more exact, let us take the case of a patient with hip degenerative arthritis. He can as well suffer from spinal arthritis too. The clinical picture is usually overlapping.

When a patient decides to have a total hip replacement operation, it is possible that pain deriving from the spine was a contributing factor too. When I had a patient of this type, I tried to explain to him this coexistence. Injecting his spine, I relieved him to some extend of his spinal problem. The pain that persisted was the one that the hip operation would help. The arthroplasty would certainly improve the spinal problem too, by restoring stance and walking. Nevertheless, he should expect in future some problems from the spine, for which he should report back. In this way I prepared my patients to return back to protect the operation I had done on them.

This is what probably happened with one of my patients. A woman, still alive, now over 90, with bilateral total hip replacement, both cemented. A metal-to-metal one side done in 1972 and a plastic-to-metal on the other side done in 1976. She lives in a town 70 miles from Thessaloniki. Over the last twenty years, she visited me from time to time, terrified, because the local doctors were telling her that she most probably needed revision. Paravertebral injections helped her, since her symptoms were mainly referred pain. Five years ago she had a revision of the hip that was done thirty seven years before. The reason was a fatigue fracture of the metal. The ball of the femoral implant was separated from the femoral stem. It was a McKee-Farrar prosthesis which the surgeon who revised the hip was kind enough to send it back to me. I still have it.

The pes anserinus syndrome may coexist with osteoarthritic knees. I believe that this is responsible for the persistence of postoperative pain after knee replacements in quite a number of cases. If one is ready to handle it before leading the patient to the surgical table, he might not have to deal with it afterwards.

One of my first bilateral hip arthroplasties had an L4-L5, 1st degree spondylolisthesis. She had heavy family obligations and had to report back quite frequently with pain round her hips, which responded to para-vertebral injections. She finally developed bilateral sinking hips. I don't know if her spinal problem had led to that. Thinking of her I still regret not having done a spinal fusion to her. Besides the fact that fusion could stop her from suffering, I wonder if it would have saved her hips from sinking.

This kind of retrospect thinking is an attempt to interpret treatment practices that I had been applying since the late sixties in regards to hips and since the eighties in regards to knees.

Facets & late Sciatica

It is not rare for someone, who had a successfully operated PID (Prolapsed Intervertebral Disk), many years ago, to report back with sciatica and intermittent claudication, on the same or the contralateral side. The Lasegue's sign is usually negative and the narrowing of disc space as well as the bulging of discs is usually reported. Once the SLR reaches 90 degrees, it makes no sense to speak about pressure on any nerve root. The facet joints, all these years, had to work in a subluxated position due to the approximation of the vertebral bodies. This had led them to wear and tear. These cases usually respond to one or two para-vertebral injections. A spasm of the nutrient vessel of the sciatic nerve is quite probably the cause of symptoms which the para-vertebral injections can release. The result was better when I had to inject the contralateral side too.

Quite often the patient points to you painful spots in muscular areas, such as the origin of gluteal muscles. On palpation they are really tender. This tenderness usually disappears straight away after injecting the facets only. The spots which require injection are those near the insertion of gluteus medius and minimus to greater trochanter and gluteus maximus to linea aspera. In many cases the relief after injecting the facets is only temporal. Maybe these are the cases where spinal fusion could offer a lot.

I have done quite a lot of operations on PID cases in the past. Having the experience of both operative and conservative treatment, I could decide in the limits of my competence, which one was best for the patients. Gradually, I became a second opinion doctor, especially for patients who were told that surgery was the only solution to their persisting problem. I must say that quite a number of them did well without surgery. I believe that it would be useful for orthopedic surgeons and neurosurgeons to get some experience in injecting the spine. This was the way I came to understand, to some extent what is really going in this territory.

The abdomen is an area where lumbar facets can play around. General surgeons, gastroenterologists, urologists and gynecologists, know that some of their problems start from the spine. I am afraid that most of them will very seldom inquire their patients about any spinal problem they had in the past and they are usually unwilling to ask their patient to turn over to examine his back. Quite possibly, they are not quite sure what they should look for.

Some examples are worth mentioning. A general surgeon and a friend of mine, asked me once to examine his secretary whose problem was a persisting meteorism. He had done all possible tests over the last two months and found nothing. Now he had turned to me, wondering if her problem could be related to her spine. He was right to suspect that, but even though he was one of the best general surgeons I knew, spine was the last thing he thought of. Actually, she had a thoracolumbar scoliotic curve. Meteorism subsided after one para-vertebral injection. My advice to the surgeon was to buy her a decent office chair.

One day, a collaborating physiotherapist, escorted his friend to my office whom he was treating for pain in his lumbar area, radiating to the anterolateral aspect of the thigh. He had reached a point where he could not help him anymore and turned to me hopping that my injections might help. The patient was an athletic young man, who after the end of the day's work, grasped his motocross bike and run to the mountains. He had a muscular spasm and tenderness at the left of the spine, at the L2 to L4 level.

Preparing for the injection I asked him if this pain had any radiation to the genitalia. He instantly looked up at the physiotherapist, who promptly defended himself by saying: "I didn't say anything". As they explained to me, he had been admitted urgently two weeks earlier in a private clinic with acute pain to his left testicle. All tests done proved nothing. Pain subsided gradually. On the fifth day he was discharged with no satisfactory diagnosis. Most probably, the urologist was unaware that he was actually handling a spinal problem.

Whenever I came across a facet syndrome, the only proof that my diagnosis was correct was the positive response to treatment. By injecting the facets and getting a positive result, treatment is already underway. This makes in most cases admission and investigation unnecessary.

For a period of seven years (1979-1986), I had a part-time appointment as a consultant to the Cancer Hospital of Thessaloniki. My job, apart from operating bone tumors and doing all sorts of bone biopsies, was to help oncologists to differentiate between metastatic and arthritic pain of the spine. Scanograms were positive to both metastatic and degenerative lesions. Para-vertebral injections, proved most helpful to doctors and patients, relieving them from unnecessary distress.

Lumbar Facets, Hip Joint and Urology

Reaching the end of this book I intend to close with a case which I believe is touching the aetiology of hip osteoarthritis. This is one of my old cases which after a gap of seven years had to return back to me. Being myself already sensitized and suspecting what facets can do, I was ready to follow this in alert, step by step all along. It is let me say a prospective study on a single case, if one is allowed to call it so. It was certainly an opportunity to recall and retrospect similar cases which although I had treated in the past, I had crossed them out just because I could not accept them to be osteoarthritic cases. I was simply not ready at that time to accept that taboo issues like hip osteoarthritis could have simple answers. I intend to return after discussing the present case, with a similar one going back to the early seventies.

This is a lumbar facet case which I have been following for the last 38 years. It concerns a male subject, a civil engineer. At the age of 26, I saw him first for a sprained ankle which was a recurrent problem for the last three years. One local injection and strapping, was all what he needed. The following year he came to see me for a low back pain. It was the result of long sitting working hours. X-rays showed nothing in particular. I told him that I would treat his back the same way I had treated his sprained ankle one year earlier, by injecting his spine now. For the next 25 years or so he was visiting me once every three years on average, to treat a relapse when the usual non-steroid drugs did not work. One injection was enough each time.

In mid-nineties he had an accident which caused to him a central transverse non-displaced fracture of the acetabular fossa. The weight bearing area remained intact. He did well keeping off weight bearing for three months. For the next 7 years he had no problem with his hip apart from a pull, as he described it, at the front of the hip joint when he had to open his pace.

Seven years later the hip which had sustained the injury started hurting. He started at the same time having micturition problems. He had difficulty urinating and a diminished flow. In spite of treatment his condition deteriorated, evolving to almost incontinence, something that terrified him. The MRI at this stage reported evidence of circulatory problem both in femoral head and acetabulum. He had to use crutches for a period of three months. Five months after the start of this present problem osteophytes appeared on x-rays round the acetabular rim. This picture got worse two months later. The joint space was not affected. His doctor told him that he was at the early stage of hip osteoarthritis for which nothing could be done to stop it and that sooner or later he would need a total hip replacement. This is the diagnosis that any orthopaedic surgeon would do.

The urologist, having tried all possible ways to help him and finding no way out, suggested that he should seek advice from the doctor who was taking care of his spine in the past for the possibility his micturition problem to be a spinal one.

He rang me then. This was the moment I regained contact with him. It was seven months after the onset of his present problem. He limped with significant pain, internal rotation at the hip joint was lost and painful, and there was tenderness in the font of the hip joint and upwards along the psoas muscle. He admitted that he had neglected his spine during the last year.

I told the patient that I must first inject his lumbar spine as I used to do it in the past and the psoas tendon as well in front, but I would not touch the hip joint itself at this stage. On our next appointment, in a week's time, we would discuss about the joint. The response to this first injection would help me to understand what exactly happens and how serious his problem is.

One week later he reported a lot of improvement on what concerns pain on weight bearing but some tenderness still remained at the front of the joint. He added that the micturition problem had also improved.

So, both hip joint and bladder were helped after injecting his lumbar facets and psoas tendon. It was reasonable for me to suspect that both these problems could have a common origin. I grasped the opportunity to discuss with my patient his problem the way I understood it. I explained to him that past experience had led me to believe that a condition known as "idiopathic necrosis of the medial femoral condyle" is caused by the spine. It is some sort of bone infarct. If this is true, that the spine can cause a bone infarct to the lower part of the femur, why not be possible that it can also affect the femoral head. I do not know it. Nobody knows. What I also do not know is if the upset inflicted on the blood supply of the femoral head, as the MRI had reported, was still reversible. The only thing I could do was to continue what I had started. In other words experiment. The MRI he would bring in two weeks' time would answer all these questions.

He agreed at once. He had nothing to lose since my colleagues had already condemned his hip and he had run out of options. At this second appointment, apart from the facets and the psoas, I injected the hip joint too. It was his improvement that encouraged me to do this. Now nobody could blame me for aggravating the situation. I felt that I had to do this. I could not ignore the possibility that some proprioceptors of the articular capsule might demand attention too.

The MRI which he brought two weeks later reported impressive improvement. The MRI which was repeated four weeks later reported full restoration to normal on what concerned the blood supply of femoral head. He had a total of four treatments, the last one on the eighth week. The intra-articular injection was done only once at his second visit.

Six months after his last treatment he was still symptoms free on what hip and bladder concerned. He had his lumbar spine and psoas tendon injected one month later for some discomfort he felt.

So, both orthopaedic and urinary problems were cured at least till the last time I saw him ten months after the start of treatment just by injecting proprioceptors. For what concerns the micturition problem, I can allege that I had come across and treated another facet syndrome since I had treated the spine only and I had done nothing aiming to help the bladder. That was an unexpected discovery. When an orthopaedic surgeon treats a urological problem then he is trespassing. In this case trespassing was unintentional. It was actually an accidental side effect of the treatment which was given to treat the orthopaedic problem.

I am well aware that most urologists know that some of their problems start from the spine. The urologist who was handling this case certainly did and so he finally acted by sending him back to me. What accidentally was revealed in this case was its exact origin and how this can be treated when it is a facet one. It is only for the urologists to speak about its frequency.

For what concerns the hip joint, things are not so simple to analyze. I cannot allege that I had treated another facet syndrome. The reason is clear. I did not inject the facets only. I injected the psoas muscle and tendon too. I infiltrated the anterior joint capsule externally and I injected once the joint internally, even though I knew and still believe that hip OA cannot be treated with intra-articular injections. Furthermore, there was the history of an injury of the same joint. My personal belief is that this joint had fully recovered from the injury and did not deserve to end as an osteoarthritic hip. As for the discomfort he felt on extending the hip joint, I always felt that this could possibly be due to posttraumatic adhesions between the anterior part of the joint capsule and the psoas tendon sheath.

Proprioceptors similar to those of the facets are found in the hip capsule, the psoas muscle and tendon. They are equally important and they have the same facilities to communicate and deliver their distress signals to any direction. Any one of them could claim to be the invisible terrorist. You can't ignore them. You have to suspect them and look till the last one of them has been satisfied. It makes no sense discussing which of them had started the problem, the lumbar facets or those round the hip joint. All of them belong to the same group. My interference in this case was infiltrating nerve receptors only. I have not done anything else. Actually facet syndromes are proprioceptors' syndromes, with the facet ones having the biggest share. Keeping the term facet syndrome for this case, I believe it makes no difference. If in the future hip OA is accepted to be another facet syndrome, then what this case tells us is that the disease may still be reversible the seventh month after its onset.

This case illustrates how the facets behave, or to be more exact, how I enjoy imagining them behave. For the first 25 years it was enough for them to display their problem with a low back pain pointing to the suffering area. From the moment they were attended properly the patient was able to return to his usual activity routine. The injury of the hip joint and the continuation of some discomfort in the area had as effect to restrict his activities. This turned to be in favor of the facets which remained quiet for the next seven years. During the last year for various reasons he neglected his lumbar facets, considering their increased grumbling as an expected consequence of the aging process.

Now the facets, considering themselves neglected, (this is where the myth starts) they decided to proceed to terrorism hoping that this way they might be heard. They picked up as targets the hip joint and the bladder using the vasomotor centers to do the dirty job for them. I do not know how far they would proceed with the bladder but I do know quite well how far they would go with the hip. At this stage the patient's and doctors' attention was concentrated on the new situation. The spinal symptoms which were still there were easily forgotten.

This case reveals also the peculiarity of facets on what concerns treatment. The usual consequence of events in medicine is first you diagnose then you decide how to treat. With facet syndromes, although the actions are the same the sequence appears to be reversed. You can only suspect that you have come upon a facet syndrome and must proceed with the treatment, expecting the diagnosis to follow a few days later as a confirmation or rejection of your initial hypothesis.

It was fortunate with this case that I had to do with an educated and sensible person. When I told him bluntly that the only possible help I could offer was to "experiment" on him, he did not hesitate to accept it. It is unfortunate though that the treatment started late. Things could have been much better if this had started 7 months earlier. May be it proved to be not too late for the femoral head since the blood supply was restored. I am not however sure if this can last since the capsule has been affected too. Now the joint proprioceptors are involved too and they should be watched in addition to the facet ones.

I will now mention a similar case, as I already promised. This has really occupied my mind over the last forty years.

It is all about a schoolmate of mine who came from my home town to see me for a problem of his hip joint. The local orthopaedic surgeons had diagnosed the onset of hip osteoarthritis and were discussing with him about surgical intervention since any treatment they had tried over the last three months had failed. The x-ray films he brought were of a normal hip joint. He walked with a limp, the joint itself was tender on palpation and internal rotation was restricted and painful. He mentioned that his lumbar spine had been painful lately.

Although I did not disagree with my colleagues' diagnosis I suggested injecting his spine for the possibility some of the pain to be a referred one from the spine and the psoas muscle. The immediate response was not satisfactory so I proceeded to infiltration of the psoas tendon and the joint itself relieving him at that moment completely from pain. I did all these just because I felt I had to do something for him. I did not really believe that I could really help.

One week later he rang me to thank me for saving his hip. Twenty years later in a reunion meeting he was still grateful. I felt really uncomfortable because I did not and still do not know, what I had really treated. It could be a psoas tendinitis but I had never come in the past across such a case so I could not be sure that this was really one. I could not accept what I had treated could possibly be osteoarthritis.

Fifty years ago, before the prevalence of total hip replacements, the intertrochanteric displacement osteotomy was the most popular choice to treat the hip OA. I remembered that some surgeons at Oswestry believed that the medial shift of lesser trochanter was the reason of the obtained relief by removing the friction of the psoas tendon on the femoral neck. If this is the case then the psoas proprioceptors could be involved in the whole process.

Rheumatoid Arthritis

I always considered rheumatoid arthritis to be a generalized collagen disease and rheumatologist the right one to treat this entity. The orthopaedic surgeon can be involved when there is need for surgical intervention to help with deformities.

This disease is rather rare in southern countries like Greece and usually appears with a lighter and more benign form. Whenever I came upon such a case I referred it to the rheumatologists. Before doing so I was taking care of the local problem by injecting the suffering joints but I insisted that the patient should see a rheumatologist because he was in need of a systemic treatment which I was not qualified to provide.

Occasionally a certified rheumatoid case was coming to me for a persisting local problem. Treating the local problem with injections the result was satisfactory and quite often permanent when seen at an early stage. I always wondered why the rheumatologists do not usually practice local injections to their patients. I believed that a few of joint deformities could be avoided if apart from the systemic treatment, the local problems were also dealt with. I was dealing with them applying the same scholasticism as with cases of Sudeck's syndrome. I did not hesitate to inject every single wrist, MP and proximal interphalangeal joint. I had again the feeling that I was breaking a vicious circle. This could be tackled only after a local intervention under the cover of the systemic one.

I have never related the facet joints with rheumatoid arthritis. From this aspect this chapter is irrelevant to this book. Never the less a rheumatoid patient can develop a facet syndrome in the same sense this could happen to anybody else. This would certainly aggravate and confuse the whole picture. This is a possibility that cannot be excluded and certainly has to be dealt with.

Exacerbations of ankylosing spondylitis, in the phase the disease is retreating, could be manifestations of this kind and they could be dealt the same way locally, not having to change the therapeutic regime the patient is already on.

Treatment

The local injecting technique is the only treatment method that I knew and applied when treating the spinal facet syndromes. All my experience is based exclusively on this and I am afraid I cannot offer advice on any other therapeutic approach.

Treating a facet syndrome, one accepts that he is handling a mechanically induced disorder. Apart from trauma, mechanical strain on facet joints might be the cause. Questioning the patient, one tries to find out what is the real cause. Once you have done this, it is crucial to make it clear to your patient that he cannot expect any improvement from your treatment unless he is ready to help, by reducing strain and avoiding actions which led to that.

At the beginning, when symptoms start as mere smoke signals from the facet region, the infiltration of the facets alone is enough. When these signals have been ignored repeatedly, for weeks or even months then the vasomotor centers take over. This is the stage where peripheral organs, nerves and vessels are affected. The treatment is useless when the latter have sustained irreversible changes.

All cases described in this book, have been classified by me as spinal facet syndromes. I could not interpret them being anything else since I had treated them successfully as such. I had to accept that the answer could be so simple. The reader should also note that I have avoided meticulously referring to details concerning routes and mechanisms involved. Using terms like smoke signals and priests conducting sacrifices was a convenient way to translate things. Creating myths was very popular in Greece long time ago when the only tools available were analysis and synthesis. Myths helped people interpret what they could not explain. Occasionally they involved a god to support the myth. They were provident enough to keep a reservation for the Unknown God for future use to back up the new myth which would take the place of the dying one. Myths proved ideal to fill the gap of knowledge.

A practitioner accepts that the end recipient in medicine is the patient. His duty is to offer the best possible treatment. If he can improve treatment techniques then this is even better. He cannot be a proper researcher. Applying treatment measures one at a time is incompatible with his psychology. The feeling of fighting against time is pushing him quite often to do many things at a time. This is actually what has happened with the case of the hip joint.

Injection treatment is an aggressive approach and certainly not free of risk. It suits more surgically trained doctors, who are familiar with handling emergencies. Injecting the cervical spine, fainting or even collapse are conditions which one must be ready to face. One injects nothing to nobody without having available soluble cortisone for IV injection, if needed.

Questioning for allergies and fainting episodes is imperative. Allergy to xylocaine was my real nightmare through all these years of practice. With time, this incidence becomes a rarity since experience helps the doctor, suspect and handle carefully a patient who is prone to react badly.

Long needles, apart from being useless, are terrifying to the patient. They could be dangerous too. A disposable syringe of 5ml with a needle 21g and 1 1/2" long was the only size I could handle effectively, treating the cervical spine. Longer needles are occasionally necessary for lumbar spine. Suction before injecting is imperative.

Surgical imaging devices usually terrify the patient. Although useful at the beginning they prove with time to be less necessary. When one has reached the point not to need them the injecting process is much simplified and more easily accepted by the patient. With the patient sitting on a couch, it takes no more than 30 seconds for each side of the cervical spine to be injected. This is actually the maximum time the patient can easily endure.

An old standing stenosis of a disc space does not mean that it is the suffering level. The stiffness of that space is compensated by extra work at the above or lower level. May be these are the levels that suffer. X-rays and MRIs will not give you information about that. Only the patient's reaction to the injected fluid can pinpoint the suffering joint. It cannot be missed. The patient will state to you strait away after your intervention on his spine that something has changed. This is a partial or full relief of pain. The insertion of the needle is not painful; it is the injected fluid that hurts. If your patient thanks you for not hurting him, this means that you have missed the target.

I must confess that treating the facet syndromes I have never felt to be the master of the game. I had always to wait to find out if I had injected the right facets. They can trick you. Not infrequently one comes to realize that the facets of the other side should be injected also. I felt happier when I had the excuse to inject both sides the same time. In these cases, when it is the cervical spine what you have injected, it is usual for your patient to complain that he has lost stability. It is xylocaine who has put out of action the balance proprioceptors. It takes ten to fifteen minutes for this function to be regained. The patient is not allowed to leave your surgery till he feels confident he can walk steadily.

There is one more thing that should be stressed. One never injects cortisone if he suspects infection. The surgical field of an arthroplasty is a forbidden place too. Injecting there could be disastrous. The routine lab and X-R tests protect the doctor from mistakes. Also, one should be always on alert for a possible metastatic disease.

Research

As you can imagine, researching this topic will not be an easy task. Facet syndromes are purely clinical entities and one requires a lot of experience to be able to diagnose them. If one is going to use the para-vertebral injections as a tool, which I personally believe to be essential, it takes a lot of time to learn how to do it properly. The ability to differentiate between local and referred pain is critical. Quite often apart from the facets, other points should also be infiltrated.

I could describe this book as a clinical research done gradually, though there was no intention or planning to be one. This is just a product of experience. I have dealt only with the start, the triggering of events and their ending which is the treatment. The intermediate and most difficult part, involving centers, routes and mechanisms should be the subject of formal research. I leave this to others. You cannot knit a pullover unless you have a start and you cannot finish it if you do not know how. From this view this book could prove useful to researchers too.

Epilogue

Medicine, like all sciences, can only be learned in practice. No matter what we were taught or how much we have read, the only thing that remains is what we have had the chance to come across, to diagnose and then to treat. The information is transformed to knowledge only if it is applied and proved to be working.

What one has read in these pages is just information. Consider it food for thought or an excuse to look into it in more detail and depth. The question is if this could be transformed to real knowledge that can be generally transferred. If a doctor for example of any specialty suspects that he is facing a facet syndrome, no one would expect him to stick a needle to his patient's neck, trying to find out if it is really so. It is equally difficult for him to find somebody else familiar with this injecting technique to help him. I believe that the General Practitioner with his global knowledge of medicine can prove to be the right one to filter all these cases and refer the patient to the right expert who can help.

I am afraid that until these difficulties are overcome, it should be expected, healthy teeth to continue to be extracted, sinuses unnecessarily curetted, congestion of the medial femoral condyle to be left to end as an idiopathic bone necrosis and orthopaedic surgeons to continue trying hard for successful total hip replacements.

Made in the USA
Middletown, DE
05 November 2026

36546172R10047